INTER

MW01531094

FASTING

How To Easily Lose Weight, Keep It
Off And Improve Your Health

By

Sandra White

Table of Contents

Introduction

Dieting is one of the more difficult ventures that any of us embark on in our lives. Most of us spend years if not our whole lives attempting to find some method of eating that allows us to finally achieve the body and level of health we all desire. Unfortunately, it rarely pans out that way.

From the moment we change our eating style, our bodies are fighting against us, desperately trying to hold on to precious energy reserves, despite that fact that this change is likely a good one. Typically, dieting leads to metabolic adaptation and a reduction of energy expenditure, which means the body is continually fighting against any attempt at change. Traditional dieting methods, unfortunately, manifest as severe restriction and frustration. Further, when weight loss is the goal, most people end up gaining all of their weight lost back and then some. That's a problem, but fortunately, there's a solution.

Intermittent fasting is one of the hottest new dieting trends in the health and fitness industry but don't be fooled, as it's much more than a pattern, rather a potential new lifestyle to adopt. What sets intermittent fasting apart from other diets is mostly that it doesn't need to be a diet at all. If you choose, calorie restriction isn't a requirement, especially if you're just looking to improve your health.

This is of course without mentioning many of the other adverse effects of traditional diets such as immense hunger, the urge to binge, potential reductions of lean muscle mass and the need to significantly alter your schedule to accommodate the diet itself. According to research and anecdotal reports, intermittent fasting may mitigate these adverse effects of dieting, potentially even abolishing them all together.

Intermittent fasting is also unique in that it works according to your schedule rather than the other way around. You decide how long and when you fast, allowing you to manipulate the diet and lifestyle to fit your needs for maximum success.

Over the course of my career, working with hundreds of individuals and observing the effectiveness of the intermittent fasting approach, it's easy for me to say that it's an effective approach to weight loss but even more so as an opportunity to free one's self from the burden of continually needing to eat and monitor such consumption. Further, the evidence regarding intermittent fasting as an effective measure for a wide range of health ailments is just too substantial to ignore.

When I first began fasting over five years ago, the idea seemed entirely foreign. For ages, the recommendation had always been to increase meal frequency. To then practice the complete opposite with fasting, of course, felt a bit strange. Fortunately, intermittent fasting turned out to be much more than just a diet, but rather a lifestyle. Once I was able to understand how comfortable and convenient the practice could be, I knew that new lifestyle approach had been adopted.

When you begin to understand all facets of intermittent fasting, you'll start to understand why this method of eating is so popular and of course, why it's worked so well for so many people.

You'll understand that you don't need to eat continuously throughout the day for energy or even at all if you're not hungry. You'll be able to understand why intermittent fasting can work according to your schedule rather than the other way around. Truthfully, you'll begin to realize what's so wrong with traditional dieting and how intermittent fasting can improve the whole process.

By continuing in this brief guide, you'll not only gain a deeper understanding of how to practice intermittent fasting, but you'll gain a deeper understanding of how and why it works, providing you with greater insight for more practical and precise manipulation of the diet. Not to mention, you'll finally be able to take control over your appetite and schedule.

If you're still not convinced, consider searching for testimonials of those who have tried and succeeded using different forms of intermittent fasting. A simple Internet search of intermittent fasting will reveal just how relevant this information is and also how insanely easy and efficient the whole process can be. There's a reason that intermittent fasting has gained a cult-like following: it works.

When you read this book, you'll gain insight into the intricacies of fasting that you might not get elsewhere. You'll understand the basics of transforming your lifestyle and how to incorporate any of the many different types of fasting into your routine. Further, you'll gain insight into many of the various benefits of fasting that extend much further than merely weight reduction or maintenance. By the end of this book, you'll have the complete list of steps required to successfully implement and manipulate an intermittent fasting method into your routine in an efficient and effective manner.

But why sit on the opportunity to change your life? Getting started is the hardest part of any new venture. Change is scary, but you've already started. The fact that you've made it this far in the introduction reveals that you're ready and eager to change. The best part is, you've already started. Don't stop now. Continue down your new path and treat yourself to a higher understanding of a dieting method that just might change your life.

The information provided in this book offers a blueprint for successfully choosing and implementing an intermittent fasting routine into your own life. Throughout this book, you'll learn about the intricacies of dieting and of course how intermittent fasting provides the most accessible route. Further, you'll learn what's necessary to take back control over your food and life. You're in charge, and it's time to take control. By learning and implementing the techniques provided in this book, it's likely that you'll be practicing intermittent fasting, not as a diet but rather a new lifestyle.

Intermittent Fasting

What Is Intermittent Fasting?

Intermittent Fasting (IF), often referred to as time-restricted feeding, is a method of eating that promotes extended periods of fasting or abstinence from food, followed by a restricted window of time to eat food. Really, the term intermittent fasting is mostly just an umbrella term for a wide range of eating methods that leverage spending significant portions of the day abstaining from food.

At first, this approach to eating sounds a bit strange and likely counterintuitive to everything you've heard about nutrition in the past, but rest assured, this method of consumption is one that has withstood the test of time, likely extending all the way back to our ancestors. For them, however, it likely wasn't a matter of trying to lose weight. It's assumed that over the course of our existence, we evolved to spend significant portions of the day without food, presumably during times that we were hunting and foraging for it.

In our current western society, however, many of us eat continuously throughout the day, primarily because we've been told it's necessary to do so. For instance, you've probably heard that breakfast is the most important meal of the day, but really, there isn't any tangible evidence to support such a claim.

It's been theorized that due to this constant consumption of food throughout the day, our bodies are continually being bombarded with nutrients, promoting growth, such as increased body fat, body weight and potentially even growth of tissue that might be cancerous (1).

Additionally, one of the most common issues in America is the prevalence of insulin resistance. Insulin resistance is an issue where the body is unable to clear sugar from the blood efficiently, which can result in obesity and even type 2 Diabetes (2, 3). It's thought that by spending significant portions of the day fasting, this act may help re-sensitize the body to insulin, thus improving insulin sensitivity and reducing the risk of obesity and other metabolic related diseases (4). Because of these possibilities, many researchers and regular people alike have adopted intermittent fasting as a potential way to reduce the impact of our eating habits from both bodyweight and overall health perspective.

As we'll get into a bit later, proponents of intermittent fasting theorize that by spending significant portions of the day fasting, this time away from food not only optimizes the weight loss process by potentially increasing fat metabolism but may also improve some serious health-related issues ranging from heart and brain related, to cancer.

Different Intermittent Fasting Methods

Intermittent Fasting is a broad term to describe various methods of fasting and eating. However, regardless of the process, to be considered intermittent fasting, the dieting approach will require extended periods of time without eating with a restricted window of opportunity to eat. Fortunately for all of us, there are many different forms of intermittent fasting that you can use as a guide or precisely as laid out. This fact is also one of the best reasons to even consider intermittent fasting.

Being able to adopt a style of eating that fits best with your current schedule is a quick route to success. Luckily with intermittent fasting, there are many different ways for you to do so.

16:8 The "LeanGains" Approach

The LeanGains approach of intermittent fasting is one of the original methods that boosted the practice into the mainstream, likely because of its ease of use and straightforward tendencies. This method of intermittent fasting includes a minimum of 16 hours of fasting, followed by an 8-hour window for eating purposes.

The LeanGains approach is typically the best option for those who exercise regularly or those with typical work schedules, looking to use intermittent fasting on a daily basis. The reasons the LeanGains approach is so popular is because the fasting and feeding schedule allows for easy incorporation into a typical routine.

For example, If you were to begin the 16 hour fasting period around 8 p.m. the end of the fasting period will come right around 12:00 p.m. the next day, which is a reasonably standard lunchtime for many working-class citizens. Further, if need be, you can just shift the fasting and feeding schedule to coincide with when you typically eat your last meal and when you usually have lunch (your first meal after the fasting period.

If you're looking for an introduction to fasting, in a way that works with your schedule, the LeanGains approach is a great starting point.

Alternate Day Fasting

Alternate Day Fasting (ADF) is a bit different from many of the other methods, just because you won't be fasting on a daily basis. Traditionally in research, this method of intermittent fasting is one of the more popular, specifically for obese individuals. The reason for this is because it allows for a significant reduction of calorie intake while minimally changing the user's schedule.

Alternate day fasting is mostly just how it sounds. On one day, users of this method eat as they normally would with no restriction. On alternate days, users severely restrict calories, consuming no more than 25% of normal calories. This is considered the fasting day. For example, if a user traditional eats 3000 calories per day, on the "fasting days" they'll only consume around 750 calories. Over the course of a 7-day period, this can create a serious energy deficit, which may be quite advantageous for very obese individuals.

This method of fasting is popular for research and obese individuals alike because you mostly only need to "diet" every other day. Allowing people to eat as usual for half of the week, makes adherence much more likely to occur.

5:2

The 5:2 approach leverages similar concepts to alternate day fasting in that the majority of the week is spent eating according to regular habits. However, with this method of intermittent fasting, you'll spend at least two days per week, completely fasting, consuming little to no calories, whatsoever.

The most compelling arguments for using the 5:2 approach is surprisingly one of the best arguments in opposition to the approach. With this method of fasting, a majority of your schedule throughout the week will remain unchanged, since you'll have the ability to eat as usual for 5 of the 7 days out of the week. Since so much of the week remains unchanged, this is typically a significant selling point. However, you also have to consider that complete fasting for 24 hours or more can be quite tricky, solely from a hunger and energy perspective.

Further, it can be quite challenging to choose which days are most appropriate to place the fasting periods. Doing so will require scheduling fasting days well in advance. Not to mention, this method can prove to be quite tricky if you have an unpredictable schedule.

Overall, the 5:2 method can apply to a wide range of people and preferences but may prove difficult to use correctly, especially on an erratic schedule.

Eat-Stop-Eat

Eat-Stop-Eat is another fasting method that incorporates occasional, full 24 hours fasts. As you can imagine, this method of fasting is not as popular as some of the other, but it provides very similar positive and negative attributes that may or may not work with your preferences and schedules. This method of fasting is most beneficial if you find the 5:2 approach of fasting to fit with your schedule. Further, by using the Eat-Stop-Eat process, you may find that you have a bit more leniency when deciding on the day or days that you'll fast.

Based on the other options available, the Eat-Stop-Eat method will work best for someone that only wants to occasionally fast and does so without a clear schedule. Further, since fasting days may be scarce, intentionally reducing calorie intake will be necessary if you hope to lose bodyweight with this method consistently.

The Warrior Diet

The Warrior diet is another daily fasting method that merely uses the upper end of fasting duration. This method is typically defined by users consuming only one, large meal per day. Usually, this equates to around 20-22 hours of fasting, followed by a seriously restricted window for food consumption.

This method of fasting lends itself very well to hectic schedules. If you're always working throughout the day and have little opportunity to eat or just don't care to be bothered with eating, the warrior diet is a great approach. However, it's important to carefully consider the ramifications of spending so much time away from food on a daily basis. If you're incredibly active, fasting for 20-22 hours may prove to be difficult from an energy standpoint.

Further, with this method of fasting, you should ensure that the quality of the meal you do it is very high, such as being rich in protein, vegetables and healthy fats. With such a limited opportunity to eat, you should ensure that you're consuming adequate amounts of each macronutrient, as well as a wide variety of foods to ensure ample micronutrient consumption.

The Warrior Diet method is quite useful and lends itself to those with hectic lives or those that don't care to eat food often.

Skipping Breakfast

Lastly, the most common form of intermittent fasting is one that many people do without realizing. That happens to be merely breakfast skipping or deciding to forgo food intake based on feeling and hunger.

Breakfast is unique in that many people place great emphasis on this meal, despite it just being another opportunity to consume calories. From a weight loss perspective, skipping breakfast may help reduce the total amount of calories you consume throughout the day, leading to reductions in body weight.

Further, if you consider other "official" types of intermittent fasting, if you skip breakfast regularly, it's likely that you're spending anywhere from 12-16 hours fasting, without even considering it. This method of sporadic fasting is acceptable as long as doing so doesn't result in excess calorie intake the rest of the day.

Different Methods For Different People

As you can tell, there is a wide range of varying dieting methods that are considered to be intermittent fasting. Fortunately, you can just use any of these methods outright, or you can use them as a starting point, manipulating the fasting and feeding period to best fit your preferences, schedule and overall desires. Regardless, there are a few different pieces of information that you need to keep in mind.

First, consider choosing a method that best fits with your current schedule or at least one you feel most confident with. For instance, immediately jumping into 24 hours of fasting can be quite a shock for many, leading to the abandonment of the diet. As we'll get into later on, progressively increasing your fasting duration until you find the optimal schedule for you is extremely important for defining what's best for you, while also ensuring that the change isn't too drastic.

Second, you need to keep in mind that regardless of the method you choose, calorie intake will still be the number one determinant of your success if you're using intermittent fasting to lose weight. Intermittent fasting has the unique ability to help us inadvertently (or intentionally) reduce calorie intake. For example, if you typically eat six meals per day and then reduce that amount to only two, it's unlikely that you'll be able to compensate for the calories you didn't consume.

When making a decision, you should choose the fasting method that you will be able to actually stick too. Also, keep in mind; if weight loss is your goal, you'll need to ensure that you're effectively reducing your calorie intake as well.

Intermittent Fasting Is Not Just A Diet

When most people consider intermittent fasting, it's usually because it's often considered to be a diet, specifically for weight loss. While that's the case, it's not an absolute necessity.

Intermittent fasting, as we've touched on already, comes in many different forms, which cater to different people and different schedules. From there, it's entirely possible to manipulate any type you decide on, to best fit your schedule and needs. For instance, if you choose a daily form of fasting, you can adjust the fasting duration according to different variables in your life, such as when you wake, work, have lunchtime and even when you exercise.

Additionally, this can be done on the fly. If one day you need to fast for only 12 hours, due to some time constraint, it's no issue to do so. For example, extending the fasting period because you need to meet a work deadline is certainly acceptable.

Intermittent fasting is unique in the sense that you can adjust the schedule and requirements of the diet to fit with your needs and schedule, rather than the diet forcing you to adapt to it.

Apart from the fact that you can tailor intermittent fasting to fit your schedule, most practitioners find that it becomes a new way of life, rather than merely a diet. Fasting, contrary to popular belief makes you feel quite right. Most practitioners find that when fasting, hunger is reduced, focus and cognitive ability have been increased and you also need not spend time throughout the day worrying about and consuming food.

Above all else, intermittent fasting is extraordinarily convenient both from a weight loss and lifestyle standpoint. Once you begin, it's quite likely that it will just become a new way of life for you, rather than just another dieting method.

General Side Effects & Safety

Generally speaking, fasting is an ancient practice that has been around for thousands of years. Only in the past few years has intermittent fasting come into the spotlight as one of the hottest new dieting trends that might work.

For the most part, intermittent fasting is widely considered to be a safe practice. For instance, many medical practitioners are studying and even recommending the diet as an additive treatment for diseases such as cancer and even cardiovascular diseases.

Regardless, most diets come with at least some potential side effects and unfortunately intermittent fasting is no different. The most glaring possible side effect of fasting would be hypoglycemia or low blood sugar. Since you're restricting nutrients, doing so is forcing the body to rely on stored reserves. If you're not acclimated to the rigors of fasting, this could pose serious issues.

Additionally, it's entirely possible that during the fasting period, you'll experience some other potential symptoms of reduced energy intake such as a headache, nausea, irritability, brain fog and fatigue. While many of these may or may not occur, it should be noted that it's a possibility.

Keep in mind as we'll touch on later, many of these side effects are only present during the adaptation period when transitioning from a regular pattern of eating to that of intermittent fasting. Fortunately, most users report a reduction of transition-related side effects within a week or two of consistent practice.

All in all, there are a few side effects associated with fasting, but they are typically short-lived. If you experience these side effects to a significant degree, it's suggested that you cease fasting and begin again once the side effects have diminished. As always, consider speaking with your primary care practitioner both before starting an intermittent fasting protocol and of course if you experience severe adverse side effects.

Why Intermittent Fasting Works

Ease Of Use

One of the biggest reasons that intermittent fasting works so well for people is that it has very high ease of use and can be easily implemented with just about any schedule or goal.

First, intermittent fasting breaks the mold of traditional eating styles in that you aren't required to eat at typical times, and you don't need to eat, even if you aren't hungry. This is without mentioning that with this style of eating, you can eat many meals or condense your food all into one. The possibilities of when and how you can eat are virtually endless with intermittent fasting.

One of the most significant determinants of success when dieting will be how consistently and how firmly you can stick to whichever diet you use. With intermittent fasting, sticking to the diet is quite easy since you dictate when and how much you eat, rather than the diet deciding for you.

A great example is in the morning. In the morning before work, many people scramble to eat something under the pretense that they need energy for the day ahead. What follows is traditionally a reasonably poor meal from a nutritional standpoint. Additionally, many people consume breakfast, only because they feel doing so is necessary, rather than because they are hungry. With intermittent fasting, you can choose to abstain from breakfast if you just don't have the time or if you just are not hungry enough.

Lastly, you can manipulate your eating schedule based on your schedule. If you need to fast until 2 in the afternoon, for example, you can adjust your fasting an eating schedule to accommodate. Overall, intermittent fasting is quite easy to use and implement, which increases the likelihood that you'll remain consistent and see results.

Calorie Intake

Regardless of the dieting approach being used, if your goal is to adjust your bodyweight (or keep it the same), results depend on energy balance. Energy balance is merely a term to describe the constant ingestion and expenditure of calories. When you exercise you expend calories, and when you eat, you ingest them.

Even though many people have found success with different methods of dieting, the research shows that by and large, success is dictated by increasing or decreasing calorie intake, based on the primary goal (5).

Consider for a moment regular eating habits. Quite often, people consume 3, full meals per day, usually intertwined with 1-2 snacks throughout the day. When you begin to restrict the amount of time that you have to eat, it becomes increasingly more difficult to make up for the calories you burned during the fasting period.

For example, if you traditionally eat breakfast, a mid-morning snack and then lunch, depending on the composition of your meals, you could be consuming upwards of 1500 calories. With an entire day of opportunity, consuming this many calories and then some isn't exactly a difficult task. However, if you restrict the amount of time that you're allowed to eat food, it becomes increasingly more difficult to not only consume the same amount of calories but also to make up for the calories that you've burned during the fasting period.

Intermittent fasting makes manipulating calorie intake almost effortless, which often allows people to change their body weight and composition with relative ease.

IF Optimizes Fat Burning

While calorie balance matters the most for adjusting or maintaining your bodyweight, if you're attempting to lose some, it's best to try and lose that weight preferentially from fat mass. Intermittent fasting is a method of dieting that may help the body optimize this process to ensure that when weight is lost, it's coming primarily from body fat.

It's theorized that extended periods of fasting simulate the same conditions that would happen if you were using a ketogenic style of dieting. Essentially this means that the body begins to preferentially metabolize stored body fat for energy, rather than relying on glucose; a primary fuel source for the body that we get from eating carbohydrates mostly. In fact, some studies show that spending moderate time fasting each day may improve favor fat metabolism over that of lean muscle tissue.

For example, in a recent review comparing studies on calorie restriction and intermittent fasting, the data indicated that when subjects restricted calories through fasting, almost 90% of their weight reduction was from fat mass. This is in comparison to studies including only calorie restriction, displaying only around 75% of bodyweight lost coming from fat mass (6). Since lean muscle tissue is so valuable, this difference could be significant over an extended period.

Based on the current research, it seems that by fasting for extended periods of time, the lack of food availability during this time creates an environment within the body that improves fat metabolism.

When you consume food, a peptide hormone known as insulin is released from the pancreas. This is quite beneficial because it helps drive nutrients such as glucose, out of the blood and into various tissues like muscle. Unfortunately, however, some theories state that elevated insulin levels reduce fat burning. Essentially, insulin signals food availability to the body, which then shuts down the release of and metabolism of fat. While this notion is theoretical, it helps to explain why those practicing intermittent fasting often find a majority of their weight loss to come specifically from body fat (7, 8, 9).

Keep in mind however that despite the potential for intermittent fasting to increase fat metabolism, to lose weight, you'll still need to ensure that you're reducing the calories you ingest.

Increased Autophagy

While you may just think of food as necessary, you also need to consider how the food and amount of food you consume influences how your body builds and repairs. Autophagy is a process within the body where cells called macrophages essentially devour and recycle other cells that are old or damaged. This is hugely beneficial because damaged cells and components can lead to many health issues, such as cancer (10, 11, 12).

One of the reasons that intermittent fasting seems to be beneficial for this purpose is that research suggests autophagy doesn't work very well in the presence of nutrients like amino acids from proteins and glucose from carbohydrates (13).

See, when you consume food, this signals food availability, which stimulates pathways in the body related to the growth of body tissue such as muscle and fat. When the body is receiving these signals, it's difficult for these macrophages to function correctly, since they would be associated with the removal of tissue from the body. Mostly, food relates to growth while autophagy relates to breaking down tissue.

When you're continually providing the body with energy, such as eating throughout the day, it's theorized that the process of autophagy is severely hampered. Thus, by spending significant lengths of time without nutrient available for growth, it's thought that this process of autophagy can work, unhindered (13).

Starting Intermittent Fasting

Plan Your Transition

Regardless of the method of eating you choose, the first thing you should always do is plan out your transition into the new style of eating. This is extremely important to do because if done correctly, your new dieting style should become your new, permanent approach to eating. Since one of the most significant determinants of success with new eating patterns is consistency, you need to have a plan of attack for just about any situation.

First, you need to realize that it's likely you've been eating according to a specific schedule, perhaps for your entire life. Most people have been indoctrinated into the idea of 3 meals a day with snacks in between. If you're leaping into the world of fasting, doing so could become quite tricky if you aren't prepared.

When planning your transition, need to consider many different variables such as which method you'll use, how you'll change your routine to accommodate this new eating style, how you'll cope with potential side effects and even what you'll do if you end up deciding that intermittent fasting just isn't for you.

If you consider changing your current eating style to match an intermittent fasting method, you need to be prepared for everything to work correctly, but you also need to account for things that won't go your way. Even though intermittent fasting is quite easy to use and employ, any significant change to your current eating habits can be both mentally and physically exhausted. You should make every effort to minimize the impact that any adverse event could have on your ability to succeed.

Establish Your Fasting Method

Your first step to transitioning into the world of intermittent fasting is to choose the method of fasting that you'll be using. Will you fast daily or only a few times per week? Do you need or want short or long durations of fasting?

It's imperative to consider this ahead of time because it will naturally become the standard for how you eat, but it will also determine how you safely and effectively transition into your new schedule. For example, the transition into a daily fasting routine will be significantly different from what you would do if you decided to use alternate day fasting or the 5:2 method.

Your first step to determining the best method for you will be to consider your preferences. For example, if you need to eat breakfast for one reason or another, you'll need to shift fasting periods to accommodate this need. In this situation, you might even consider not using a fasting approach to nutrition. It's imperative that you determine these bits of information ahead of time rather than changing your routine to find out it doesn't work well for you.

It's vital that you consider your preferences such as how you typically respond to lack of food. If you find that long periods of time in the morning without eating makes you irritable or nauseous, it may then be in your best interest to adjust your fasting schedule to accommodate an earlier meal. If you exercise, for instance, will also be a driver of which method you choose and should be considered.

Once you've begun to consider your preferences, you should then attempt to find a method that works best with your current routine. This is very important especially with fasting because significantly drastic changes to your eating patterns will reduce the likelihood that you'll remain consistent and will make adhering to the new plan much more difficult.

For example, if you love to eat breakfast, then adopting a dieting pattern that revolves around skipping breakfast probably isn't the best idea. If you love to eat carbohydrates, it's probably best to avoid extreme carb restriction.

Further, you can also use this opportunity to understand how you can manipulate any intermittent fasting routine to best fit with your current routine. For example, if you typically can't eat your first meal until 2 p.m., you can just shift the fasting schedule forward two hours to accommodate. If you're using the 5:2 fasting method, you could decide to place the fasting days on days in which you are most busy.

Regardless of the decisions that you make with regards to fasting schedules, you should always try closely match the method of fasting to fit within your current routine and schedule. Doing so limits the amount of change you're going through at any given time, which makes consistency all the more convenient.

Define Your Overall Goals

After you've established which method of fasting is the best fit for you, you need to consider then precisely why you're using intermittent fasting. This information could include whether you're looking to lose weight, gain weight or even maintain weight. Further, this decision could also include the use of fasting for health-related purposes such as improving heart health or even using it as a means of life extension.

Whatever purpose you have for using intermittent fasting as your new approach to eating, defining this purpose ahead of time is very important because it will drive how much you eat and of course, what you eat once the fasting period is over with.

If you're considering intermittent fasting as a method of adjusting your body weight and composition, you'll need to ensure that you're appropriately manipulating energy balance. Energy balance is a concept that helps us manage calorie intake based on the desired result.

For example, if you're using intermittent fasting to lose weight, you'll need to ensure that you're creating a negative energy balance on a daily basis. This means that you'll need to ensure that your body is burning more calories than you're ingesting through food. Fortunately, intermittent fasting makes this process quite simple, but it's a point that needs to be considered. Many people believe that intermittent fasting provides weight loss without reducing calories. While it's a nice idea, it's one that unfortunately doesn't pan out in the real world.

If you're interested in using intermittent fasting but don't care to reduce calories, there's nothing wrong with doing so. However, since restricting calories can occur without any effort while using intermittent fasting, it's essential that you understand this. Many people have used a fasting protocol only to lose weight when weight loss was not intended accidentally. In this situation, you'll have to consider how you'll go about maintaining your current calorie intake.

Lastly, if you're hoping to gain weight, doing so will require that you eat just above your usual amount of calories. Further, when doing so, you'll also need to consider the duration of your fasting period. Since more extended fasting periods mean shorter eating periods, reductions of the fasting period may be required to ensure that you're eating enough food to gain weight.

If you're using fasting as a means of life extension or other health benefits, using just about any form of fasting that fits best with your schedule will be appropriate. However, you'll then also need to consider how you'll adjust the actual content of the food you eat if you haven't already.

Defining the reasons that you're switching to intermittent fasting is extremely important because that decision not only will drive the form and duration of fasting that you'll be using, but it will also drive how you eat after the fasting period has ended.

Change One Thing At A Time

No matter the dieting approach that you decide to use, it's essential that you don't change too many variables at once. Doing so includes switching to fasting, using a long fasting duration, incorporating exercise and even improving your nutritional habits.

Making drastic changes overnight is the easiest way to fail. Consider the overwhelming amount of people that embark on New Year's resolutions, only to abandon them after a week of change. Don't be fooled; the same situation could happen to you if you change too much or just aren't prepared for the change that will occur.

This is especially true for intermittent fasting since there is a slight adaptation period, where hunger and fatigue are genuine risks. If you put dietary restriction and exercise on top of changing to a fasting routine, the chances of success are a bit reduced.

The best way to transition into a fasting routine is wait until you've established a new habit of fasting and eating before you consider changing your food intake and incorporating exercise. This period could be anywhere from a few days to a few weeks. These changes will largely depend on how you feel, your preferences and how consistent you can be with sticking to the change.

Start With A Short Duration

Just as immediately changing everything at once can set you up for failure, so too can jumping right into a fasting routine and fasting for the full duration as laid out by which every method you choose. For example, if you've decided to use the 16:8 version of fasting or even the 5:2 method, immediately jumping into those durations of fasting can be extremely difficult.

When beginning a fasting protocol, the best option is always to ease you into the change. Switching from an eating style that allows constant consumption to a method that encourages long durations of fasting is an easy way to become hungry, irritable and eventually abandon the new eating style.

If you've chosen to use a daily method of fasting such as 16:8 or the Warrior Diet, beginning with a 12-hour fasting period as a maximum is an excellent idea. The reason for this is mainly because it's possible you're already fasting for 12 hours, without thinking about it. When you consider that most people eat dinner around 6-8 and then don't have breakfast until 8 a.m. or later, it's entirely possible that you accomplish 12 hours of fasting without even considering it.

Second, having only a slightly longer duration without food compared to your regular routine is likely to make any potential side effects much less apparent. For example, if you usually wake up and eat breakfast, when transitioning into a fasting routine, you could merely extend your regular fasting period (the time it takes from your last meal to when you eat breakfast) by 1 hour.

One additional hour added to your routine is exceptionally applicable and accomplishable. By easing yourself into fasting like this, you can help to mitigate any of the potential adverse effects of fasting such as hunger and irritability.

From there, just increase your fasting duration as you see fit. If you found that 12 hours was too long, then attempt to stick with 12 hours until it becomes comfortable. If 12 hours was relatively easy and you feel confident enough to continue, increase as you see fit. Test the waters with an additional 30 minutes of fasting each day or increase by 1 hour until you find your sweet spot.

Keep in mind that this process is also a great way to determine which method and duration of fasting is best for you. Planning things out on paper is certainly beneficial, but sometimes you won't know for sure until you try. Not to mention, this method can help you figure out how different ways or approaches to eating influence how you feel and how successful you are.

For the other forms of fasting such as 5:2, Eat Stop Eat and Alternate day fasting, you need to consider easing yourself into these durations of fasting.

Protocols such as 5:2 and Eat Stop Eat promote full 24-hour fasting periods. The issue with jumping immediately into 24-hour fasting windows is that doing so is difficult. It's likely that for most of your life, you've consumed food daily. To all of a sudden remove an integral part of your life can manifest into real issues, which could lead you to abandon the diet altogether.

The truth is, 24-hours of fasting is demanding. It can lead to significant hunger, brain fog, irritability and potential headaches. It's imperative that you realize this before beginning because it's in your best interest to be prepared for the worst, but also so that you can make smart decisions about easing your way into long durations of fasting. If you don't prepare, the chances of you abandoning fasting after one long fasting period is quite high.

When choosing a daily fasting routine, the best step you can take is to begin with 12-14 hours. The reasons for this suggestion are the same as for daily fasting. By starting with a short duration and easing yourself into longer durations, you'll help avoid many of the common mistakes while reducing the possibility of severe side effects setting in. As you become more comfortable, increase the duration as you see fit.

Keep in mind though, if you choose a method that has many days in between fasting periods, it's possible that side effects will still be present. As we'll get into in later chapters, intermittent fasting does have an adaptation period where side effects can be prominent. With extended periods without fasting between fasting days, this adaptation could be prolonged.

Alternate Day Fasting is a bit different from the other styles because, on fasting days, you'll still consume some food at around 25% of normal calories. Essentially, ADF is like the Warrior Diet (one reasonably large meal at the end of the day) completed, every other day. Even though you're still consuming some food, you're still severely restricting the amount you can consume. As such, you should again ease your way into this style of routine.

If you've decided on Alternate Day Fasting, the best option is to decrease calorie intake on the fasting day sequentially. For example, on fasting day 1, you can reduce usual calorie intake to 75% of average calories. To put into perspective, if you usually consume 2000 calories per day, on the first day of ADF, you'll consume only 1500 calories. From there, reduce by an additional 25% on each successive fasting day until you reach your desired amount.

Regardless of the method you decide on, sequentially increasing your fasting duration from a reasonably short period is the best move you can take to introduce this new eating schedule into your routine. Just remember that there is no one size fits all approach and you can undoubtedly manipulate any of these methods of fasting to fit your personality, needs and schedule.

If you're introducing yourself to the 16:8 method and find that 14 hours is your sweet spot, then you should leverage that. If when introducing yourself to alternate day fasting, you find that you're better off consuming 50% of normal calories compared to the traditional ADF routine of 25%, then so be it.

Don't get caught up in sticking to a specific schedule because it's typical. If you find that a tweak to any of these methods works better for you, then that's the best choice you can make. Fortunately, easing your way into a new fasting routine can help you make this decision alongside helping you to avoid some of the most common side effects of fasting.

Be Willing To Adjust

One major issue with how many people view dieting is that once you decide on a particular style of eating, you have to stick to it regardless of personal preference or based on your experience. For example, when given a meal plan, many people feel that unless they stick to the meal plan exactly, they won't see results. Fortunately for all of us, this is simply not the case.

When you're first beginning a new dieting approach, this is a great time to start figuring out which aspects of the diet you prefer and which aspects of the diet just aren't for you. Perhaps you've chosen a duration of fasting that's just too long or even too short. Maybe you've decided that a daily fasting regimen is more advantageous than full fasting days, twice per week.

When it comes to having successful weight loss, being able to remain consistent with both the dieting style and calorie reduction is imperative. Even more so, if you've adopted intermittent fasting solely as a means of adjusting your routine, you should adapt whichever style you choose, to best fit with your schedule and needs. If you're always miserable because of some aspect of the diet you've chosen, then you should reconsider or at least adjust the diet to reflect your needs.

If you are beginning a particular style of dieting and even a specific subset of intermittent fasting, it's imperative that you shape the diet to fit within your needs, given that you're still using the dieting method as initially intended. While small adjustments such as the duration of fasting or when the fasting period begins are probably acceptable. However, if you manipulate the diet so much that it no longer becomes fasting, then you should reconsider your overall decision and find a diet that is more suitable for your needs.

Lastly, when you're initially testing the waters and determining how to manipulate the diet for your own needs, this is a great opportunity to decide that intermittent fasting isn't for you.

We live in a world where a simple Internet search will provide you with thousands of different diets that cater to as many different personalities. If you find that fasting just isn't right for you, it's best to switch early on before you radically change your schedule and eating patterns. Remember that the most successful diet will be one that you can consistently stick to.

If you're always fighting the diet style or feel miserable all the time, then it might be a smart move to reconsider using intermittent fasting as your primary eating approach.

Understand The Adaptation Period

While intermittent fasting is quite easy, IF approaches can often be radically different from typical eating patterns and schedules, which means that there may be a slight period in which you'll experience some adverse side effects. This is known as the adaption period and is typically nothing to be concerned about since many of the issues related to fasting usually subside within a week's time. But it's imperative that you understand the real possibility of experiencing these issues so that you don't abandon the diet prematurely.

Common side effects you might experience include fatigue, headaches, hunger, mood swings, nausea, brain fog and light-headedness. It's possible that one or more of these side effects may be severe or even not present at all. Individual experiences may differ.

Of the side effects mentioned, hunger is easily the most common issue that people experience when beginning a fasting protocol, and that's to be expected. Consider for a moment that for your entire life, you've mostly eaten similarly. Chances are for most of your life you've consumed breakfast, some mid-morning snack, lunch, another snack, dinner and then maybe another snack. When you adopt a fasting routine and immediately remove breakfast, mid-morning snack and maybe even lunch, it's not entirely surprising that you'd become hungry during that time.

The reasons for this seem to mostly because hormones that control hunger such as ghrelin seem to work according to the schedule that you usually eat. Ghrelin is a hormone, secreted by cells within the gut that is released in accordance with when you typically eat. Ghrelin stimulates hunger, but it also influences the brain to cause you to get up and forage for food. If you have a reasonably steady eating schedule, ghrelin is released before your regular eating times, which once released, results in hunger (14, 15).

When you're adopting a fasting routine, these cells are still operating according to your traditional schedule. So for some time, even if you aren't eating, your stomach still secretes this hunger hormone. And unfortunately, if you don't satisfy this secretion of ghrelin, the result will be hunger and sometimes-intense hunger.

Fortunately for IF practitioners, however, these cells seem to be entrainable, meaning that they will adjust secretion schedule based on whichever schedule you provide it. Just know that doing so will require consistency to ensure that these cells adopt the new schedule. This is one of the main reasons that a progressive increase of fasting time is suggested. Within a few day's time, you can slowly increase fasting time, allowing these cells to adapt. By doing so, you potentially avoid any significant bouts of extreme hunger and possibly other side effects as well.

Overall, it's essential that you understand that there may be a slight period where you just don't feel right. Keep in mind however that this period does not last forever and the duration of this adaptation period will largely depend on your consistency and diligence in following whichever routine you've decided to pursue.

This adaptation period is the time in which most people abandon intermittent fasting. Just know that any of these side effects are not forever. After the adaptation period, many people find that intermittent fasting is quite easy and makes them feel even better than before they started. Preparing yourself for this period will ensure that you're able and ready to deal with it in the most appropriate ways.

For a smooth, natural transition into whichever intermittent fasting method you've chosen, it's highly recommended that you sequentially increase the fasting period to gradually expose yourself to what fasting is. Further, by doing so, it's likely that any side effects that you do experience will be quite small and manageable.

Best Practices For Intermittent Fasting

Adjust Around Your Schedule And Preferences

As we've touched on a few times throughout this book, the ability to adopt a new eating schedule, such as intermittent fasting will mostly rely on how smooth the transition is and how consistent you can stick to the new diet. For example, if you need to eat breakfast then using a dieting style that encourages skipping breakfast might not be the greatest idea.

On the schedule side of things, many different variables need to be considered. First, you need to ensure that whichever method of fasting you've chosen works with your current schedule. For instance, do you require breakfast in the morning because your job is physically intensive? Will you have the ability to eat most days around the scheduled end of your fasting period? These are genuine questions that you need to answer so that you can seamlessly integrate fasting into your current routine.

Second, you need to consider if your fasting schedule will also fit into your family's schedule if you have one. Consider for a moment how well fasting will work for you if the bulk of your fasting period comes during usual dinner time for your family. Chances are, things won't work out very well in this situation.

By manipulating your fasting schedule around your current schedule, it's entirely possible that you can incorporate a fasting routine into your daily life with little to no adjustment. However, if you begin to change your schedule significantly to fit within the parameters defined by the diet, it's likely that you'll run into problems.

When adopting a new eating schedule such as fasting, it's always best practice to avoid radically changing your lifestyle unless your health depends on it. If you're using intermittent fasting for moderate weight loss attempts or to receive the potential health benefits, recognize that radically changing your routine is not the best idea from a practical and consistency standpoint.

By molding the diet around your current schedule, you'll feel less of a burden and will be more likely actually to stick to the new routine.

Establish Habits That Help

Intermittent fasting can sometimes be difficult, specifically because many of the habits that you currently have, function well with your old style of eating. This includes things like when you eat, what foods you eat and also what you do throughout the rest of the day. These habits help to define how your body responds to food availability and the lack of food.

Just as with any other diet, establishing habits that help you remain consistent will be of the utmost importance. Perhaps you drink coffee in the morning to wake up and also stave off hunger. Maybe chewing gum is your answer to morning hunger pangs. Whichever tools you use to make intermittent fasting more of a lifestyle rather than a habit will only improve your experience and overall success.

Lastly, it's vital that you reevaluate any of your previous or current habits, as many of them may pose issues for a successful transition into the fasting lifestyle. For instance, eating junk food regularly may not be the best choice from a nutrient perspective when using a restricted window of time to consume food, or maybe you get a mid-morning snack each day at work.

Together, these habits can create issues with consistency and ease when fasting. It's imperative that you reevaluate current habits and adjust to fit in with your new lifestyle and routine. For example, you could transition that typical mid-morning snack to be a mid-afternoon one. While many habits will need to be changed, it's possible that many of them simply need a small adjustment rather than an entire overhaul.

Establishing habits and adjusting previous ones to fit with your new lifestyle and routine will be of the utmost importance for a successful transition into an intermittent fasting approach.

Understanding Hunger

When taking on a form of intermittent fasting, it's imperative that you understand hunger, what it means for you and how to deal with it. Being able to deal with hunger in a number of different ways will be essential for a successful transition into this style of eating. Further, you'll need to be able to delineate between acute hunger pangs and actual hunger that is related to appetite.

As mentioned earlier, when you first begin fasting there is somewhat of a transition period, which also includes when and how intensely your hunger appears. Frankly, this makes sense. If you've been consuming breakfast for your whole life, it stands to reason that you might become hungry during those periods of time that you would regularly be eating. Fortunately, this type of hunger is expected, meaning you can equip yourself to deal with it before starting the diet.

What unfortunately then becomes an issue are erratic hunger pangs. Everyone has experienced them before but understanding how to deal with them while fasting is essential. The main problem with this type of hunger is that it can result in people abandoning their fasting routine, despite the fact that their hunger was relatively minimal.

This type of hunger can occur for some different reasons, but one of the best theories for this is erratic eating behavior. As mentioned, cells that secrete ghrelin act according to a regular schedule of eating. For example, if you consistently have your first meal of the day around noon or lunchtime, then you can expect that these cells will secrete ghrelin in anticipation of this standard meal.

If you're consistently eating at strange times that differ from the day prior, it's entirely likely that the schedule of ghrelin secretion becomes influenced. When this occurs, it's entirely plausible that you'll become hungry at strange times.

If you find that you're having hunger pangs at strange times or during the fasting period, it's suggested that you first begin to establish a schedule of exactly when you eat and do not eat. By doing so, you help to train these cells only to secrete the hunger hormone, ghrelin around when you'll be able to eat. Additionally, doing so can help you rule out other potential reasons for feeling so hungry.

Second, before you decide to break your fast, attempt to have some water. While it's possible that you may be dehydrated, the water you consume may help stretched stomach cells, reducing hunger.

Third, consider improving the quality of your food. Since the window of time available for you to consume food is small, it's possible that you're just not eating enough or not eating enough of the right types of food. In this case, it's suggested that a majority of your food intake leans towards lean protein and fibrous vegetables. Protein and fiber both help to slow digestion and improve satiety, which can prove to be extremely valuable from both a hunger and body composition standpoint.

Lastly, if you simply cannot deal with hunger, it's best to consider how you can manipulate the diet to fit your needs. For instance, perhaps you need to shorten the fasting duration or need to reduce the days that you fast. Maybe you find that you need to shift your fasting schedule to a different time of day. All of these variables could be influencing your hunger and should be considered.

The truth is that with any diet, including intermittent fasting, being able to delineate between acute hunger pangs and real hunger and appetite will help you to be able to control cravings better and of course, overall calorie intake.

Consistently Practice Your Diet

When it comes to new diets, many people want some form of quick fix. There's no denying that a new diet idea that preaches natural weight loss seems like a quick fix, but rarely does it ever pan out as such. Intermittent fasting is no different. find success, you'll need to use this method of dieting as often as possible to begin to change not only your body but also your mindset.

First, whichever method of fasting you decide on, it's crucial that you remain consistent, ensuring that you're practicing your diet in the same way as often as possible. If for instance, you decide to use a daily form of intermittent fasting, it's always a good idea to try and use that method of eating daily, including the weekends.

Many people like to think of dieting as a weekday only event. This often results in practitioners using the diet-style on Monday through Friday, just to completely abandon it throughout the weekend. If you want to be successful, this is not suggested.

One of the main reasons that you should stick with the diet 7 days a week is because fasting relies heavily on your schedule. Interestingly enough, ghrelin-secreting cells also are dependent on a schedule. Those cells secrete this hunger hormone based on circadian rhythm, meaning that they work according to your typical schedule of when you eat and do not eat (14, 15).

Theoretically, this is one of the most persuasive arguments for why people using intermittent fasting don't experience extreme hunger. Since during the fasting period, there's no stimulus to cause a release of ghrelin, which means you don't get hungry.

If you're using an erratic eating schedule, however, it becomes much more difficult for these cells to begin adapting to the new schedule, mostly because there isn't one. Just as your energy levels are optimized when you sleep and wake at similar times each day, the same concepts hold true for your nutritional protocol.

If you've chosen a method of fasting that is not daily, this poses a few unique issues that you'll need to consider. Since you're not fasting daily, it becomes a bit more difficult for the body to adapt to the schedule. When you fast daily, the body can respond since it "believes" this is the new schedule. However, when you're spending 3-5 days in between fasting days, the signals provided to the body may not be strong enough to promote a real adaptation.

In this case, it's strongly suggested that you at least attempt to maintain some schedule. This could mean fasting on the same days each week and ensuring that the number of days between fasting days is consistent. By doing so, you'll increase the likelihood that your body adapts to the new schedule, potentially growing ease and effectiveness of the new diet.

Just remember that the more consistent you are with your practice, the quicker you'll adapt and the easier your new diet will be to stick to. If you're always changing with an erratic schedule, using intermittent fasting may prove to be quite tricky. By maintaining a consistent schedule, it's likely that practicing IF will be a much smoother process.

Use Stimulants Like Coffee & Green Tea

While most foods and beverages are considered forbidden when fasting, most practitioners of the eating style agree that the fasting period is a great time for using stimulants such as caffeine from coffee.

Fasting promotes the release of what are known as catecholamines. Catecholamines are hormones that are released from the adrenal glands in response to some form of stress. This stress can be fear, anxiety, stress itself and of course, fasting.

When you begin fasting, the lack of nutrient availability increases the output of these catecholamines, such as epinephrine, norepinephrine and cortisol. Interestingly enough, when this occurs, it can lead to improved cognition and potentially even improved fat burning from stubborn fat areas (16, 17).

Interestingly enough, stimulants such as caffeine also encourage the output of these hormones, such as norepinephrine (18). Thus, when fasting, it's entirely possible that you'll be able to leverage these hormones both from stimulants such as caffeine and even fasting itself. Apart from the apparent cognitive benefit of increasing caffeine and these hormones, elevating levels of hormones like norepinephrine may have a positive and powerful influence on hunger (19).

Additionally, there is even evidence to suggest that beverages such as coffee may possess other attributes that can significantly influence hunger. For instance, in a recent study, researchers tested the influence of both regular and decaffeinated coffee on different measures of hunger.

In this study, researchers placed subjects into three different groups. The first group consumed caffeine in water, group two drank caffeinated coffee and group three consumed decaffeinated coffee. During this study period, researchers then measured the amount of a hormone known as peptide YY.

Peptide YY is a hormone that is released in the gut in response to food intake. From there, it then acts on different regions of the brain to signal reduced appetite. Thus, increasing the level of this hormone in the body is quite advantageous for reducing appetite and managing hunger (20).

Interestingly enough, in this study, the researcher's determined that consuming decaffeinated coffee increased levels of peptide YY to the most significant extent, with regular coffee coming in second. This means that while caffeine itself may positively influence appetite, it's possible that there is some other ingredient in coffee that acts independently to reduce hunger, making the fasting period much more manageable.

Additionally, if you're not precisely interested in drinking coffee, considering green tea may be a viable alternative. Interestingly, green tea holds the ability to also increase catecholamines like the ones promoted through coffee intake. Even more, green tea also provides antioxidants known as catechins, with a special one in particular known as EGCG.

What's so exciting is how green tea influences catecholamines and their action in the body. Like coffee, green tea contains natural caffeine. This caffeine is then able to stimulate the release of catecholamines, which not only improve fat loss but may also help to reduce appetite.

Interestingly though is how the EGCG catechin interacts with these hormones. Traditionally, once catecholamine levels rise, this is met with an increase of an enzyme called catechol-O-transferase; otherwise known as COMT. This enzyme acts to break down these catecholamines. Interestingly enough, evidence suggests that the EGCG catechin acts to inhibit the breakdown of these hormones, allowing them to remain in circulation (21).

In addition to the potential appetite suppression that these catecholamines afford us, there is also evidence to suggest that increasing these catecholamines may improve cognition, such as being able to consolidate memories into long-term memories. Fundamentally, not only can using these ingredients strengthen your fasting experience but doing so while fasted may also improve cognition and overall memory (22).

When you're fasting, if you're not extremely sensitive to stimulants such as coffee or green tea, making use of these ingredients can be extremely advantageous for reducing appetite and potentially even cognition. Further, this fantastic research suggests that even consuming decaffeinated coffee may positively influence your appetite, even if you're too sensitive to stimulants. If you find that you're having issues with appetite or feel a bit of brain fog and fatigue, a simple cup of coffee or green tea might just do the trick.

Dealing With Your Environment

Adjusting and dealing with your environment is an often-overlooked variable that must be accounted for.

Consider for a moment how tempting different environmental cues can be regarding hunger. If you work in an office, perhaps co-workers bring in "less than healthy" treats of maybe your teammates like to get burgers each day late in the morning, before your fast ends. In these situations, you'll need to understand how to adapt so that you don't abandon your diet or even better yet, how you can manipulate your diet to accommodate the environment.

Being able to avoid temptation is a real issue, especially with new diets. We see other people enjoying food whenever and however they want, and by doing so, it tempts us to do the same.

Preparing for this instance ahead of time is extremely important for success. For example, if your co-workers regularly bring in high-calorie foods for everyone to enjoy, you can pre-establish a limit of consumption or bring in a different snack for your consumption.

If you work at a job with typical lunchtimes, you can certainly adjust the beginning of your fasting period to accommodate. For example, if you practice a 16:8 fasting routine and your co-workers typically eat lunch around 11:00 am, you can just shift your fasting period to start an hour earlier than usual for instance. On the food side of the equation, you can also choose to bring your meals or choose healthier options from the menu.

Fortunately, at home, you have much higher control over the temptations that are placed in front of you. In this situation, you can mold your environment to fit your needs. For example, if you have a bad habit of eating cookies daily, you can stop buying them or restrict yourself to once or twice per week. Further, you can also decide how food is displayed to you. If you find that snacks displayed on the counter are just too tempting, you can choose to remove them.

Your environment you're in plays a significant role in the temptation you have and how quickly you'll be able to remain consistent with your new routine. It's imperative that you adjust your environment to fit your needs or adjust your habits to fit within your environment for success.

Stay Hydrated

One of the more obvious suggestions is that you should ensure that you remain hydrated both during and after the fasting period. It's safe to say that staying hydrated is essential for life. However, being hydrated also means that for the most part, the body can work optimally. In fact, research suggests that the volume of cells, or the size and amount of water each cell is holding, significantly influences how they function (23).

Further, maintaining constant hydration during the fasting period is of the utmost importance, primarily because it can sometimes be challenging to maintain hydration. During the fasting period, you're spending much of your time not thinking about consuming food and beverages. As a result, forgetting to hydrate is often commonplace when fasting.

Regarding health, avoiding water consumption for hours on end can prove to result in adverse health effects, especially if you're practicing something such as fasting. According to the Mayo Clinic, when adults become severely dehydrated, this status can manifest in different side effects such as a headache, dizziness, and fatigue (24). Unfortunately, many of these side effects can come from fasting alone, so avoiding compounding effects of dehydration is imperative.

In a similar matter, water consumption can be a powerful tool for managing hunger both during the day and with meals. As mentioned earlier, the cells within the stomach are sensitive to stretch. This is one of the mechanisms through which your body recognizes that you've eaten food, reducing hunger signals. Fortunately, water does the same thing. When you ingest relatively large quantities of water, this helps to stretch the stomach, potentially reducing feelings of hunger. As a result, if consumed before a meal, doing so could significantly reduce calorie intake as well.

Interestingly, research corroborates this idea. In a recent research experiment, scientists had middle-aged subjects placed on a diet. However, one of the groups was provided with 500ml (~2 cups) of water, before consuming full meals. What they found was that when subjects drank water before meals, these individuals consumed significantly less food and lost 44% more body weight than groups not consuming pre-meal water beverages (25). Considering that the only difference in success was water consumption, these findings can be significant.

While on the surface it seems that consuming water regularly would only be advantageous for weight loss, this technique can also be quite beneficial for those merely practicing fasting for health benefits. Even when weight loss is not a primary objective, hunger still becomes a side effect that must be managed. This information lets us understand that water can mitigate hunger without having to break the fasting period.

When fasting, it's imperative that you maintain a system of regular hydration to avoid accidental dehydration. Further, regular consumption of water can be a meaningful tool for reducing any potential side effects of fasting, such as hunger.

Keep Busy

A great feature of IF is that you can avoid thinking about food during your most productive and busy times. No longer will you need to break your essential task mid-morning to grab a snack.

When you fast, it's always best to attempt to keep your mind distracted. This is why most choose to have the bulk of the fasting period at night and while at work. By doing so, you keep yourself distracted, avoiding any tempting thoughts about food or perhaps about the fact that you're hungry.

If at all possible, consider placing your fasting period during a time in which you're busy and pre-occupied. Doing so will likely help improve your fasting experience while helping you avoid thinking about hunger.

Ensure Proper Sleep

One of the other more apparent suggestions is that you maintain a proper sleep schedule. Regarding optimal health, getting adequate sleep each night is beneficial for more reasons than one. But when you're fasting, you need to realize that sleep can become one of your most powerful tools for success.

At least when you're first starting out, lack of food availability can result in immense fatigue if not managed properly. By ensuring that you get adequate rest, you reduce the likelihood of becoming fatigued from lack of sleep and energy availability at the same time.

Second, you should also consider how lack of sleep could negatively influence your food choices. In fact, recent research suggests that inadequate sleep can result in significantly higher energy intake at meals, which can then result in excess weight gain and further, keep in mind that this research does not include the variable of fasting (26).

Lack of sleep can certainly result in extreme hunger, especially during the fasting period. Not to mention, the potential for over-consumption of food is already somewhat elevated with fasting alone. Combining fasting with inadequate sleep and the risk of over-consuming calories and the results could be downright disastrous.

Lastly, consider that sleep plays an integral role in circadian rhythm. Having regular sleep and wake times is imperative for optimal body function and regulations of many different hormones, especially those associated with energy metabolism and hunger (26, 27). By maintaining a healthy and appropriate sleep schedule, you can potentially begin to optimize how your body functions. If you're exposing the body to an erratic schedule, adapting to a fasting protocol can prove to be quite tricky.

It's always appropriate to have a healthy sleep and wake schedule. Adding intermittent fasting to the mix makes that requirement all the more legitimate. It's suggested that you attempt to get at least 7-8 of high quality sleep each night. The duration of which you choose to sleep will be mostly subjective.

Manipulating Calories

Regardless of the reasons you have for choosing intermittent fasting, you need to manage your calories appropriately. While intermittent fasting makes weight loss quite easy, it can also present issues if you aren't interested in losing weight or wish to gain some.

Intermittent fasting has the unique ability to help those who practice it, reduce calories with relative ease, which makes weight loss quite simple. By restricting the amount of time available to consume food, it becomes increasingly difficult to compensate for the calories that were expended during the fasting period. This is one of the main reasons why most find success with fasting if weight loss is a goal.

If then you're making the decision to use fasting for health benefits and don't care to lose weight, you need to have a system in place to ensure that you're consuming enough calories to maintain your weight. Remember that weight largely depends on energy balance or the ratio of calories that you're consuming relative to the calories that you're expending. If you hope to maintain your weight or increase it, you'll need to match your calorie intake to your expenditure or increase calorie consumption, respectively.

Lastly, even though intermittent fasting can help you reduce calories with ease, using this method of eating is not a free pass to consume any and all foods you desire. If you're constantly breaking your fasts with extremely high-calorie foods, it can become quite easy to accidentally over consume calories, relative to your body's energy requirements.

For the most part, intermittent fasting can make reducing calories quite easy, but if weight loss is not a goal, this can present issues. Depending on your level of commitment and intention, it's suggested that you attempt to moderate your calorie intake through one avenue or another.

Breaking The Fast

When breaking the fast, it's essential that you do so by consuming a quality meal comprised of a hefty dose of each macronutrient. Since you've spent a significant portion of the day without sustenance, it's always best practice to consume a high-quality meal at the first chance you get.

The composition of the meal that you consume after the fast will largely depend on your preferences, but for the most part, it should be a meal that is quite high in protein. The exception to this will be if you practice a ketogenic style of dieting, in which your meal would be fat based.

Regardless, since you've spent a significant portion of the day without nutrients, it's important that you provide your body with an ample amount of high-quality nutrients, rather than opting for something of lower quality. It's suggested that you stick with a meal primarily focused on some form of lean protein, fibrous vegetables and potentially some form of complex carbohydrate. While one meal won't make or break your progress, it's crucial that you choose ingredients that are nutrient dense, especially since the window of opportunity to eat is shortened.

In the long run, the composition of single meals is relatively irrelevant, but it's always good practice to maintain a high level of quality food intake, especially when using a fasting method. By having high-quality meals after the fast, you ensure that even with a shortened time window to eat, you still consume the nutrients that you require to function and thrive.

Exercise & Fasting

As a part of any healthy lifestyle, exercise should always be considered. However, if you're planning on using intermittent fasting along with an exercise routine, there are a few things you need to keep in mind as well as some best practices for ensuring safe and effective exercise in conjunction with your fasting protocol. Further, exercise can also be a powerful tool for helping you get through the fasting period in multiple ways.

Exercising Fasted

Exercising during the fasting period is a hotly debated topic and whether or not you decide to do so, will largely depend on your ability and personal preference. Some people prefer to exercise on a full stomach, while others prefer to have little or no food available when exercising. The choice to do so will be yours.

However, keep in mind, as we'll get into later that exercising fasted may change how you feel and of course, your performance. For example, you may find that if you're a runner, you have less endurance when running fasted. If you find something like this to be true for you, you should consider the ramifications of such a decrease in performance and how that will influence your schedule.

Many people enjoy training fasted while others find doing so to feel almost impossible. Doing so will largely depend on your personal preference.

Understand Changes

When you first begin a fasting protocol and are continuing to exercise, you need to be acutely aware that performance may or may not be drastically different from when you were eating as usual. Remember that your body adapts to its environment, which means benefits you've received from exercise may also rely on the food you eat.

For example, many people choose to exercise in the mornings. If you've been exercising on a full stomach in the morning and have now adopted a fasting method that has you fasting until mid-afternoon, this could significantly impact your performance.

Further, you'll need to consider any potential adverse effects of fasting. If you feel lightheaded or fatigued during the fast, it might not be in your best interest to attempt to exercise on top of that. Just understand that your performance ability may be drastically different once you adopt a fasting lifestyle and you should adjust accordingly.

Re-Assess Your Ability

As mentioned, it's likely that your performance will change once you begin fasting. As such, it's in your best interest to re-assess your ability by easing your way back into exercising.

By slowly reincorporating exercise into your routine, you'll begin to have an understanding of whether or not fasting has positively or negatively influenced your performance and to what extent. Doing so is imperative for avoiding injury. It's suggested that you pay close attention to your ability and then adjust your exercise sessions accordingly.

Adjust Your Fasting If Needed

If exercising is an integral part of your life, then it may be in your best interest to change your exercise schedule or change your fasting schedule to fit your needs. For example, if you prefer to exercise in the morning, it may be beneficial for you to shift the beginning of the fasting period to come earlier in the day. As a result, you can place the end of the fast to coincide with the end of your exercise session, for instance. Alternatively, you may find that it's a better idea for you to exercise around lunchtime or later in the afternoon, once the fasting period is over with.

Realistically, you should determine which variable is more important to you. If fasting is more important than exercise, change your exercise routine to fit your fasting needs. If exercise is most important, then it's best practice to manipulate your fasting to accommodate your exercise.

Exercise Nutrition While Fasting

What is acceptable to eat around exercise is a common question when it comes to fasting. Truthfully, the type of food you consume or if you consume anything at all will largely depend on personal preference.

However, keep in mind that when exercising, it's important to attempt to have some form of nutrition around the workout. This can mean consuming some form of amino acids before, during or after exercising. When exercising, you need nutrients such as amino acids to recover. Consuming some form of protein around the workout helps to ensure that you're actually receiving the nutrition necessary to reap the benefits of exercise.

If your exercise session comes towards the end of your fasting period, it's always suggested that you consume some form of protein, such as whey or a plant-based equivalent. If you are unable to exercise on a full stomach, it's then suggested that you consume some form of branched-chain amino acid (BCAA) supplement. Both of these ingredients provide amino acids to ensure that muscle can recover and grow from the rigors of exercise.

If your exercise session must be completed during the fasting period for one reason or another, the decision to consume some form of protein will largely depend on why you're fasting in the first place.

If, for example, you're fasting for health benefits outside of weight loss, it's suggested that you keep calorie intake low or non-existent. The health benefits such as increased autophagy and insulin sensitivity rely heavily on the absence of food signaling. Unfortunately, even a simple BCAA supplement can be enough to stop these processes. As such, consuming anything around your workout in this situation is not advised.

Your decision to consume or abstain from nutrients around the workout will largely depend on your purpose for fasting and your overall preference. In the grand scheme of things, if you prefer to have whey protein or amino acids around your workout while you fast, doing so will probably only have minimal influence on your success. Regardless, if possible, consume a high-quality protein source either before, during or after your exercise session for proper recovery.

Exercise May Help Reduce Appetite

If you've decided that exercising while fasted is acceptable or even the right move, you should also consider how exercising can influence your hunger, making the fasting period both more natural and overall more effective.

In fact, one recent study exposed obese individuals to different exercise protocols to observe its effect on hunger and appetite. Interestingly, when these obese individuals were exposed to 4, 30-second sprints, doing so significantly reduced hunger while inhibiting the release of the hunger hormone known as ghrelin (28).

The best part of this is that these individuals sprinted according to their ability. Often in research like this, individuals are exposed to study protocols that are way too intense, relative to the subject's ability. When this occurs, most of the data that results is meaningless. This is largely because it's difficult to translate the results into what might happen in the real world. If subjects are exposed to demands that they can't handle in the real world, it's unlikely the results will have any relevance.

Fortunately, these individuals sprinted according to what they could do, and no more. Based on these findings, it's clear that short, intense exercise can have a meaningful impact on reducing hormones such as Ghrelin and of course, helping to reduce appetite altogether. It's strongly advised that if you're struggling with hunger during the fasting period, consider occasionally completing short, yet high-intensity bursts of exercise. Doing so may allow you to better deal with fasting-associated hunger.

Just always keep in mind that fasting may negatively influence your performance. It's strongly advised that you remain well hydrated while also paying close attention to your ability and how you feel. If you feel fatigued, lightheaded or nauseous other than as a result of exercise, it's strongly advised that you cease exercising and reconsider your ability while fasting.

Dealing With Social Gatherings

Dealing with social gatherings while attempting to maintain a healthy lifestyle is often easier said than done. This is mostly in part because most social gatherings, whether large or small, don't accommodate those on diets. For instance, most big parties have traditional party type food like pizza, hotdogs, burgers and perhaps even cake. In these situations, sticking to your diet can be easier said than done.

Also, you also need to consider what happens when you're placed in a social situation with food that happens to fall during your typical fasting period. In this case, you'll have the choice to continue avoiding food or to break the fast. Truthfully, this decision will be based on many different variables that will ultimately come down to your own decision.

There's no denying that breaking the fast prematurely may disrupt your schedule, but on occasion, doing so won't be the reason for success or failure. Life will sometimes cause disruptions to your regular schedule, which will require you to pivot and that's okay.

When dealing with these sorts of situations, it's important to consider which variable is more important to you. Is maintaining the fasting routine of the utmost importance or do you feel that a little indulgence will benefit you? Making this sort of decision will be entirely up to you, but you should at least consider the ramifications of whichever decision you make.

Just keep in mind that you want your diet to accommodate your own life rather than the other way around. It's suggested that you avoid sacrificing events and gatherings at the hand of remaining consistent with your diet.

What is Acceptable And Not Acceptable While Fasting

What you can and cannot consume during your fasting periods will largely depend on the form of fasting you're using, the intent of which you are using intermittent fasting for and of course, your personal preference.

Calorie Consumption

Fasting, by definition, means that you're consuming almost nothing of caloric value for an extended period. The reason for this is quite simple. When you consume things that have calories, this signals growth in the body, which is different from what fasting is meant to promote. For instance, the benefit of increased autophagy afforded by fasting will be significantly diminished if growth pathways in the body are stimulated due to consuming nutrients (13).

Second, if a goal of yours is to improve insulin sensitivity, almost all calories will need to be avoided. While carbohydrates are the typical macronutrient that stimulates a release of insulin, protein also is a potent stimulator. In this case, if you're hoping to improve insulin sensitivity, it's suggested that you consume nothing of caloric value.

If you are fasting for health purposes, it's suggested that you consume little to no calories whatsoever during the fasting period, with the exception of black coffee or tea. Otherwise, you'll be completely defeating the purpose of fasting in the first place.

If you are using intermittent fasting to improve body composition, the lines between what you can and cannot consume are a bit blurred. This is in part because most people choose to consume some form of calories around the workout. If your exercise session happens to fall during the fasting period, you will have to decide whether or not progress from exercising or the potential benefits of fasting are more important.

If you decide that consuming some food around the workout is a requirement, it's suggested that you attempt to consume the minimum of whatever ingredient you choose and the ingredients should be limited. For example, a good choice in this situation would be to consume whey or a plant-based alternative just prior to or after your workout. If however, you cannot tolerate full shakes while your workout, a BCAA supplement is then suggested.

Just keep in mind that this suggestion should be utilized only around the workout. If you consume these ingredients throughout the fasting period otherwise, then you're probably not fasting at all.

If you need to question whether or not a particular ingredient is acceptable during the fast, there is a good chance that it isn't. It's suggested that you stick to beverages that contain little to no calories whatsoever. Further, if you do need to consume nutrients, such as protein around a workout, it's suggested that you keep those events to a minimum.

Potential Mistakes & How To Avoid Them

When beginning any new dieting method or approach, there are often mistakes that are made that could be easily avoided by having foreknowledge and a plan of action. Fortunately, many of the common mistakes associated with fasting are easily handled.

Fasting Too Long, Too Quickly

Easily, the biggest mistake people make when beginning a fasting routine is fasting for far too long, right from the start. This is often partly due to motivation but also a lack of understanding of how fasting will influence your body.

Keep in mind that it's likely you've been eating according to a fairly regular routine. After years and years of exposure to this schedule, the body becomes optimized according to it. Just as you can sleep and wake at the same time each day, much of the rest of the body works in a similar fashion according to your typical schedule.

When beginning a fasting routine, you need to first have a plan for how to transition and what to do when it doesn't go according to plan and second, you need to ease yourself into your new routine. A good suggestion is to begin with a modest fasting duration of around 12 hours, with much of the fasting period occurring while you sleep. This for example, would mean fasting from 8 at night until 8 in the morning. Once you feel comfortable, attempt to extend the duration of the fasting period by thirty minutes to one hour until you find the most appropriate fasting duration for you.

By using this duration, you'll gradually expose yourself to longer periods of fasting, while avoiding some of the negative side effects of fasting too long, too soon.

Consuming Too Many Calories

Another mistake many make with fasting is accidental consumption of excess calories. It is true that fasting makes calorie reduction quite easy, but just because the time available for you to eat is shortened, doesn't mean that you can't over consume calories.

If you find that you've gained weight with fasting, it's entirely possible that you're consuming too many calories. In this instance, it's extremely important that you first adjust the foods you're eating and then consider calorie tracking.

Consuming high-calorie dense foods can create issues because they have little impact on hunger and satiety, yet still provide large amounts of calories. For example, walnuts are often considered to be quite healthy. However, just one cup of walnuts is approximately 800 calories, providing 80 grams of fat. If you believe that foods such as nuts are quite healthy, it's possible that you could be consuming the equivalent of two cheeseburgers worth of calories, without even realizing it.

It's suggested that you at least pay attention to the foods you're eating, placing a primary emphasis on high quality, low calorie dense, and nutrient-dense foods such as lean protein, fibrous vegetables and complex carbohydrates.

Not Manipulating Calories

If you're using intermittent fasting for weight change purposes, it's strongly advised that you continue to pay attention to calorie intake. When it comes to modifying bodyweight, adjusting calories should be your number one focus. Unfortunately, many people have the idea that intermittent fasting alone, without calorie restriction, leads to significant weight loss. The evidence simply does not agree.

If you're attempting to lose weight via intermittent fasting, you should continue to monitor your calorie intake, regardless of the method you use. If you aren't actually reducing calorie intake, then you won't see the results you desire. Just don't get pulled into the trap of think that the diet alone is what is causing weight loss. Rather, the diet simply makes calorie restriction easy, which often results in weight loss.

Keep in mind that this scenario also deals with weight and muscle gain. If you're using intermittent fasting to improve body composition, you need to understand that this method of dieting may make it difficult to consume large amounts of food if you require it for progress. In this case, you'll need to monitor your food intake to ensure that you're consuming adequate calories. If not, you should consider adjusting the fasting period to accommodate.

Not Staying Consistent

Consistency is key with just about any diet. However, it seems that consistency is even more important when using an intermittent fasting routine, primarily because of how the body responds to schedule.

Many of the different aspects of intermittent fasting rely on a typical schedule. For example, those ghrelin secreting cells in your stomach, which regulate hunger, act according to your typical schedule. If you're constantly eating and fasting at erratic times, it makes it quite difficult for the body to adapt.

Regardless of the method you choose, it's strongly advised that you create a routine that you can stick to on a daily basis for the most optimal results.

Potential Benefits Of Intermittent Fasting

General Benefits

While intermittent fasting is often considered to be a weight loss diet, new and fascinating evidence is beginning to emerge, showing us that this ancient practice may actually provide benefit outside of simple weight loss. Even though many of these benefits are health related, there are also a few that might inadvertently improve your life.

More Time For Productivity

One of the most apparent benefits of fasting is greater time availability throughout the day to focus on productivity and other important tasks. Consider for a moment how much time you spend with food each day. For the most part, consumption of meals takes anywhere from 15-30 minutes, further, that's not including the time it takes to actually make the meal itself.

By spending much of the day fasting, the time you originally spent cooking and consuming meals can now be used for other, more important tasks. Before you know it, you could afford yourself multiple hours of free time, within a week's time of consistent fasting throughout the morning.

Improved Cognition

Many users of intermittent fasting report that doing so actually improves cognition. Fortunately, research corroborates this idea. As we've discussed earlier, fasting promotes the release of catecholamines such as epinephrine and norepinephrine. These hormones can then enter the brain and stimulate what is known as our sympathetic nervous system. Interestingly, the sympathetic nervous system regulates energy and alertness levels, which can significantly improve cognitive ability.

In fact, in one study when mice were exposed to a normal eating pattern of an alternate-day fasting routine, mice that fasted displayed significantly improved learning ability as well as overall memory (29). This could translate to meaningful improvements of cognitive ability in humans if practiced regularly.

Keep in mind that much research with regards to intermittent fasting and cognition is in its infancy. Whether fasting improves your cognitive ability will largely be subjective.

Easy Weight Loss

One of the most glaring benefits of intermittent fasting is that weight loss typically comes with relative ease if practiced regularly. This is mainly due to the restricted time availability to consume food. What most people find is that having a limited amount of time to eat makes compensation of calories lost during the fasting period, quite difficult.

From a calorie perspective, having 8 hours to consume food seems fairly reasonable. However, you must consider the effect that food has on you and your body. For example, if you consume a meal comprised of a large amount of protein and fibrous vegetables, it's possible that you won't be hungry again for a few hours.

Because of this lack of hunger and high level of satisfaction, many people find that forcing them to eat is the only way to consume adequate calories.

Second, intermittent fasting paradoxically reduces hunger. This seems largely due to how ghrelin secreting cells function. Since they release ghrelin according to when you typically eat, the fasting period all but abolishes hunger signals such as this. With no food present, there's nothing to initiate the release of ghrelin (14, 15). Theoretically, this is one of the major reasons why people experience reduced hunger when fasting. Fortunately, this makes weight loss attempts quite easy.

Lastly, one specific benefit of fasting is that the practice seems to target body fat specifically. In multiple studies in humans with daily and alternate-day fasting, these subject displayed reductions of fat mass, while maintaining lean muscle mass. Whereas most diets simply target weight loss, intermittent fasting may specifically help you lose body fat, which can be quite beneficial (30, 31).

Advantageous For Social Gatherings & Nighttime Events

One of the most underutilized benefits of intermittent fasting is that using this method can allow you to indulge when at social gatherings and large events.

If for example you have a party later on in the day and know that food options will be less than healthy, you can choose to simply continue fasting as normal, or even extend the fasting period based on the level of indulgence you plan to participate in.

Keep in mind that weight gain is largely due to the total amount of calories that you consume. If you're concerned about potentially consuming too many, you can choose to fast before or afterward to help compensate for the extra amount of calories that you're consuming.

Alternatively, if you're attending gatherings or large events that occur during the day, regular bouts of fasting will help prepare you to spend significant portions of the day without food. While your colleagues spend time worrying about and finding food, you'll be freed up to work or enjoy the gathering as desired.

Leveraging fasting allows you to indulge from time to time with little concern of ruining your progress, simply because you can make up for the mishap with slightly extended periods of fasting.

Health Benefits

In addition to general benefits and weight loss, intermittent fasting may also provide some other potent, health-related benefits that warrant its use. Reports of fasting improving brain and cardiovascular health, improved insulin sensitivity and glucose control and even potential uses for cancer and cardiovascular disease are all par for the course. As it turns out, fasting may be one of the most beneficial dieting styles in existence.

Cardiovascular Health

As it turns out, intermittent fasting may hold attributes that help to improve cardiovascular health for many different individuals. This is in part due to intermittent fasting's ability to help individuals reduce calorie intake, which often results in additional benefits in terms of heart health.

Hypertension

Otherwise known as high blood pressure, research on intermittent fasting reveals that for the most part when subjects are placed on a calorically restricted diet, using an intermittent fasting approach, and these individuals display reductions in blood pressure. For example, in a 2003 study, researchers revealed when rats were exposed to intermittent food deprivation (intermittent fasting), they displayed significantly lower heart rate and blood pressure at baseline. What's more is that they also displayed significantly lower increases in these two variables when exposed to stressful stimuli (32).

In a different study where subjects were exposed to short-term fasting (1-2 days), researchers found that this short duration of fasting was quite effective in improving markers of heart health. In fact, the results showed that almost 82% of individuals that participated in the short fasting period displayed significantly lower blood pressure, into ranges that would be typically considered to be of a healthy range (32, 33).

Based on these findings, it's fairly clear that intermittent fasting may hold attributes that positively influence heart health. Further, it's also possible that calorie restriction at the hand of fasting may also be partly responsible. However, it seems that occasional fasting of varying durations may actually positively influence blood pressure.

Heart Health

While most research regarding intermittent fasting and heart health focuses on other variables that may influence the health of the heart itself, (such as hypertension) there is emerging evidence to suggest that intermittent fasting may actually improve the function of the heart itself.

In fact, in a recent study, researchers displayed that when rats were placed on an intermittent fasting regimen, subjects displayed significantly lower inflammation and an increase of an event known as apoptosis; otherwise known as programmed cell death (34).

While that sounds scary and bad, it's a natural and necessary part of our body's health. When cells in the body are damaged or unneeded, if not dealt with, the cells can produce inflammation and even damage other cells. Fortunately, most cells are programmed to die in these instances. Once these cells have been killed, processes such as autophagy occur to recycle to garbage components.

This study showed us that intermittent fasting might help to reduce harmful inflammation while also encouraging apoptosis of unneeded and damaged cells. Together, this combines to improve overall heart health and function.

Insulin Sensitivity & Glucose Tolerance

Insulin sensitivity and glucose tolerance help to describe how our bodies handle different nutrients once they are digested. For example, if you're insulin sensitive, the body can handle the nutrients you provide with relative ease, even if you're consuming large amounts in one sitting.

When you consume nutrients like protein and carbohydrates, the nutrients begin to break down and enter the bloodstream for various uses. In particular, when carbohydrates are consumed, they are broken down into the simplest form of sugar, known as glucose. From here, glucose then enters the bloodstream for many different purposes. Once it enters the bloodstream, the glucose triggers the release of a peptide hormone known as insulin. Insulin then shuttles this glucose out of the blood into various tissues. Just remember that glucose does have a few potential routes it can take.

First, glucose can be used immediately if needed, such as if you were participating in an athletic event. If unused, the remaining glucose then gets shuttled to different organs and tissue such as the liver and muscle for storage in a form known as glycogen. Afterward, if all other outlets have been exhausted, glucose can then be transported to fat tissue and converted into triglyceride through a process known as De Novo Lipogenesis (35).

Unfortunately, if carbohydrates are consistently being consumed in significant amounts, despite low activity, this leads to a disorder known as insulin resistance.

Insulin release is relative to the amount of glucose entering the blood and the speed at which it enters the blood. For example, if you consume a piece of white bread or drank some sugar water, that high amount of sugar will enter the blood very quickly, stimulating a fast and significant insulin response. While on occasion this is nothing to be concerned about if done regularly, multiple times throughout the day, it's possible to develop insulin resistance; a condition where the body no longer responds to insulin, meaning blood glucose levels remain consistently high.

Unfortunately, this disorder has been considered to be a number one cause of obesity and metabolic disease, which comes with a host of other issues (36, 37).

Interestingly, research shows us that regular periods of fasting may improve insulin sensitivity and how the body handles glucose. In fact, in one study, researchers had subject practice intermittent fasting for 20 hours, every other day, for 15 days. Upon completion of the study, these subjects were exposed to a device known as a euglycemic clamp.

A euglycemic clamp is a constant infusion of glucose, directly into the blood. The objective of the clamp is to keep blood glucose steady and by doing so, researchers can determine how well insulin is working to drive glucose out of blood. Essentially, if more glucose is needed to maintain blood glucose levels, that means that insulin is functioning well. For instance, if insulin is working, then it will remove glucose from the blood with relative ease, meaning more glucose is needed to maintain a constant level.

Interestingly, these researchers showed that just 15 days of alternate day fasting significantly improves insulin sensitivity, which could be extremely meaningful for individuals that might happen actually to be insulin resistant (38).

Current theory suggests that because intermittent fasting includes prolonged periods of time without food, this window of opportunity provides the body with time to allow insulin-secreting cells to recover, in effect, improving its ability to shuttle glucose out of the blood.

Cancer

While intermittent fasting indeed won't act as a standalone treatment for cancer, many are beginning to consider the dieting practice as a potential additive treatment. It's thought that intermittent fasting helps to improve cell health, while encouraging the removal of damaged cells that may pose issues, through the process of autophagy.

Other research suggests that the use of intermittent fasting alongside chemotherapy may protect non-cancerous cells. Unfortunately, chemotherapy medication is formulated to cause cell death, and for the most part, these drugs are unable to distinguish between healthy, standard cells and deadly cancerous ones.

Fortunately, in one case study, researchers showed that regular, short-term fasts, lasting around 48 hours before chemotherapy was effective in reducing chemotherapy side effects such as fatigue, weakness and digestive issues. Further, in combination with fasting and reduced side effects, there was no apparent reduction of chemotherapy success, which means that fasting is at least a plausible additive to reduce the impact of chemotherapy in cancer patients (39).

Other research suggests that fasting diets may help to slow progression of cancer after it's already become established. In fact, one study showed that when chemotherapy treatment was combined with a fast-mimicking diet, actually increased levels of immune cells known as CD8 tumor-infiltrating lymphocytes.

While that may sound a bit wild, these cells enter tumors to kill and starve the cells. Fortunately, it seems that these lymphocytes preferentially target tumor cells, leaving normal, healthy ones to flourish. As a result, these researchers believe fasting might prove to be a new standard, complementing established chemotherapy treatments (40).

Based on findings such as these, fasting is beginning to be revealed as much more than a simple fat loss diet. If used correctly in combination with other established treatments, intermittent fasting may help reduce side effects of cancer treatment and even act as an additive treatment, potentially slowing the progression of these issues or possibly also preventing them from occurring in the first place.

Brain Health & Function

Surprisingly, intermittent fasting may prove to be useful for improving cognition and potentially brain health as a whole. As it turns out, fasting acts as a form of stress on the body. By reducing nutrient availability, this forces the body to adapt.

Interestingly, the stress that fasting places on the brain stimulate the release of a growth factor known as BDNF, otherwise known as brain-derived neurotrophic factor. What's so amazing about this is that BDNF protects and may even promote the growth of neurons, or nerves that transmit information throughout our brain and bodies. Additionally, it's thought that BDNF also plays a role in dealing with stress, memory, attention and even how well neurons communicate with one another (41, 42, 43, 44, 45).

New and exciting research on intermittent fasting is revealing that its effects may extend much further than pure weight loss or health benefits, but may be extremely integral in maintaining and promoting future brain health.

Inflammation

Inflammation is a relatively broad term that's thrown around quite often. However, it's a severe condition that should not be avoided if you're looking to improve health.

Inflammation merely is an immune response, which if left unchecked, may lead to severe complications. When the body is stressed, such as through exercise, the result is an inflammatory response to fix any damage. Since the muscle tissue may have been slightly damaged as a result of exercise, the body responds by sending white blood cells to the affected area to help improve recovery. Telltale signs of inflammation such as red and irritated skin or soreness then often accompany this.

While that acute response is entirely necessary and appropriate, many individuals have chronic, systemic inflammation in which the body begins attacking healthy tissue. Unfortunately, causes of this type of inflammation are often unknown, but can sometimes be due to dietary choices. Fortunately, studies show that regular intermittent fasting might help.

As it turns out, recent research corroborates this idea. One study showed that when subjects partook in Ramadan, the Muslim practice of daily fasting, subjects displayed significantly reduced markers or pro-inflammatory cytokines. These cytokines are signaling molecules, which result in inflammation. By reducing their ability to propagate throughout the body, the resultant inflammatory response may be diminished (46, 47).

Conclusion

Intermittent fasting is considered to be a weight loss diet, but most practitioners find that once they've implemented fasting into their lives, it's so much more than a mere tactic to lose weight. Fortunately, many different forms of fasting cater to just about anyone's schedule, whether sedentary or active.

Interestingly enough, this is one of the leading selling points of intermittent fasting. It's a convenient method of eating that allows you to manipulate based on your schedule and preferences rather than forcing you to adapt to the diet itself. As a result, you get a method of eating that's convenient and makes the process of managing calories almost second nature.

Intermittent fasting is useful for both weight loss and weight management primarily because of its ability to allow you to manage calories with ease.

Placing restrictions on the amount of time you have to eat makes compensating for burned calories during the fasting period quite tricky. Fortunately, this means that manipulating calories for weight loss can be quite simple and effective.

Although, IF is so much more than just a way to manipulate calories. Because of the nature of fasting, it's also convenient for most individuals. Whereas traditional diets preach the importance of consuming breakfast and increasing the frequency of meal consumption, intermittent fasting allows you to decide for yourself. If you're not hungry in the morning, fasting allows you to skip it. In doing so, intermittent fasting gives you the power to decide what and how you consume food.

Keep in mind; intermittent fasting is not without its potential downsides. While intermittent fasting is an ancient practice that is widely considered to be safe, fasting is typically a radical change compared to previous eating habits. Switching to this method of eating overnight can present issues that may attempt to thwart your attempts at reform. Because of this adaptation period in which side effects are possible, sequential transitioning into this style of dieting is a must. After slowly incorporating fasting into your routine, you'll be able to manipulate the diet to fit your preferences and schedule.

In addition to intermittent fasting's ability to change body composition, new and exciting research is emerging, showing us that fasting's benefits extend much further than weight loss alone. New research suggests that fasting may hold unique benefits that positively influence different aspects of our life, including disease. While IF is often used for weight loss, this research indicates that it may provide powerful life extension and disease prevention and treatment qualities that can be leveraged.

Together, these positive benefits create not only a diet but a potential new lifestyle that can improve your ability to manage food intake while also potentially improve various markers of health. Intermittent fasting has the potential to become a new way of life that might positively influence your life. So then, let me ask. Why haven't you started yet?

References

1. Huang, S., & Houghton, P. J. (2003). Targeting mTOR signaling for cancer therapy. Current opinion in pharmacology, 3(4), 371-377.

2. Greenfield, J. R., & Campbell, L. V. (2004). Insulin resistance and obesity. Clinics in dermatology, 22(4), 289-295.

3. Taylor, R. (2012). Insulin resistance and type 2 diabetes. Diabetes, 61(4), 778-779.

4. Halberg, N., Henriksen, M., Söderhamn, N., Stallknecht, B., Ploug, T., Schjerling, P., & Dela, F. (2005). Effect of intermittent fasting and refeeding on insulin action in healthy men. Journal of applied physiology, 99(6), 2128-2136.

5. Spiegelman, B. M., & Flier, J. S. (2001). Obesity and the regulation of energy balance. Cell, 104(4), 531-543.

6. Saltiel, A. R., & Kahn, C. R. (2001). Insulin signaling and the regulation of glucose and lipid metabolism. Nature, 414(6865), 799.

7. Muoio, D. M., & Newgard, C. B. (2008). Fatty acid oxidation and insulin action: when less is more. Diabetes, 57(6), 1455-1456.

8. Lamming, D. W., & Sabatini, D. M. (2013). A central role for mTOR in lipid homeostasis. Cell metabolism, 18(4), 465-469.

9. Sidossis, L. S., Stuart, C. A., Shulman, G. I., Lopaschuk, G. D., & Wolfe, R. R. (1996). Glucose plus insulin regulate fat oxidation by controlling the rate of fatty acid entry into the mitochondria. The Journal of clinical investigation, 98(10), 2244-2250.

10. Mizushima, N., & Komatsu, M. (2011). Autophagy: renovation of cells and tissues. Cell, 147(4), 728-741.

11. Seyfried, T. N. (2015). Cancer as a mitochondrial metabolic disease. Frontiers in cell and developmental biology, 3, 43.

12. Choi, K. S. (2012). Autophagy and cancer. Experimental & molecular medicine, 44(2), 109.

13. Liu, H. Y., Han, J., Cao, S. Y., Hong, T., Zhuo, D., Shi, J., ... & Cao, W. (2009). Hepatic Autophagy is suppressed in the presence of insulin resistance and hyperinsulinemia inhibition of FoxO1-dependent expression of key autophagy genes by insulin. Journal of Biological Chemistry, 284(45), 31484-31492.

14. Sakata, I., & Sakai, T. (2010). Ghrelin cells in the gastrointestinal tract. International journal of peptides, 2010.

15. Lesauter, J., Hoque, N., Weintraub, M., Pfaff, D. W., & Silver, R. (2009). Stomach ghrelin-secreting cells as food-entrainable circadian clocks. Proceedings of the National Academy of Sciences, 106(32), 13582-13587. doi:10.1073/pnas.0906426106

16. Chan, J. L., Mietus, J. E., Raciti, P. M., Goldberger, A. L., & Mantzoros, C. S. (2007).

Short-term fasting-induced autonomic activation and changes in catecholamine levels are not mediated by changes in leptin levels in healthy humans. Clinical endocrinology, 66(1), 49-57.

17.   Waterhouse, B. D., Moises, H. C., Yeh, H. H., & Woodward, D. J. (1982). Norepinephrine enhancement of inhibitory synaptic mechanisms in cerebellum and cerebral cortex: mediation by beta adrenergic receptors. journal of Pharmacology and Experimental Therapeutics, 221(2), 495-506.

18.   Papadelis, C., Kourtidou-Papadeli, C., Vlachogiannis, E., Skepastianos, P., Bamidis, P., Maglaveras, N., & Pappas, K. (2003). Effects of mental workload and caffeine on catecholamines and blood pressure compared to performance variations. Brain and cognition, 51(1), 143-154.

19.   Guilland, J. C., Moreau, D., Genet, J. M., & Klepping, J. (1988). Role of catecholamines in regulation by feeding of energy balance following

chronic exercise in rats. Physiology & behavior, 42(4), 365-369.

20. Batterham, R. L., & Bloom, S. R. (2003). The gut hormone peptide YY regulates appetite. Annals of the New York Academy of Sciences, 994(1), 162-168.

21. Gugler, R., & Dengler, H. J. (1973). Inhibition of human liver catechol-O-methyltransferase by flavonoids. Naunyn-Schmiedeberg's archives of pharmacology, 276(2), 223-233.

22. McMorris, T. (2016). Developing the catecholamines hypothesis for the acute exercise-cognition interaction in humans: lessons from animal studies. Physiology & behavior, 165, 291-299.

23. Häussinger, D. (1996). The role of cellular hydration in the regulation of cell function. Biochemical Journal, 313(Pt 3), 697.

24. Dehydration. (2018, February 15). Retrieved February 27, 2018, from https://www.mayoclinic.org/diseases-

conditions/dehydration/symptoms-causes/syc-20354086

25.   Dennis, E. A., Dengo, A. L., Comber, D. L., Flack, K. D., Savla, J., Davy, K. P., & Davy, B. M. (2010). Water consumption increases weight loss during a hypocaloric diet intervention in middle-aged and older adults. Obesity, 18(2), 300-307.

26.   Monk, T. H. (1991). Sleep and circadian rhythms. Experimental gerontology, 26(2-3), 233-243.

27.   Leproult, R., Holmbäck, U., & Van Cauter, E. (2014). Circadian misalignment augments markers of insulin resistance and inflammation, independently of sleep loss. Diabetes, 63(6), 1860-1869.

28.   Holliday, A., & Blannin, A. K. (2017). Very low volume sprint interval exercise suppresses subjective appetite, lowers acylated ghrelin, and elevates GLP-1 in overweight individuals: a pilot study. Nutrients, 9(4), 362.

29.   Li, L., Wang, Z., & Zuo, Z. (2013). Chronic intermittent fasting improves cognitive functions and brain structures in mice. PloS one, 8(6), e66069.

30.   Varady, K. A. (2011). Intermittent versus daily calorie restriction: which diet regimen is more effective for weight loss?. Obesity reviews, 12(7).

31.   Varady, K. A., Bhutani, S., Klempel, M. C., Kroeger, C. M., Trepanowski, J. F., Haus, J. M., ... & Calvo, Y. (2013). Alternate day fasting for weight loss in normal weight and overweight subjects: a randomized controlled trial. Nutrition journal, 12(1), 146.

32.   Wan, R., Camandola, S., & Mattson, M. P. (2003). Intermittent food deprivation improves cardiovascular and neuroendocrine responses to stress in rats. The Journal of nutrition, 133(6), 1921-1929.

33.   Goldhamer, A. C., Lisle, D. J., Sultana, P., Anderson, S. V., Parpia, B., Hughes, B., & Campbell, T. C. (2002). Medically supervised

water-only fasting in the treatment of borderline hypertension. The Journal of Alternative & Complementary Medicine, 8(5), 643-650.

34.   Longo, V. D., & Panda, S. (2016). Fasting, circadian rhythms, and time-restricted feeding in healthy lifespan. Cell metabolism, 23(6), 1048-1059.

35.   Wan, R., Ahmet, I., Brown, M., Cheng, A., Kamimura, N., Talan, M., & Mattson, M. P. (2010). Cardioprotective effect of intermittent fasting is associated with an elevation of adiponectin levels in rats. The Journal of nutritional biochemistry, 21(5), 413-417.

36.   Acheson, K. J., Schutz, Y., Bessard, T., Anantharaman, K. R. I. S. H. N. A., Flatt, J. P., & Jequier, E. (1988). Glycogen storage capacity and de novo lipogenesis during massive carbohydrate overfeeding in man. The American journal of clinical nutrition, 48(2), 240-247.

37.   Greenfield, J. R., & Campbell, L. V. (2004). Insulin resistance and obesity. Clinics in dermatology, 22(4), 289-295.

38.   Resnick, H. E., Jones, K., Ruotolo, G., Jain, A. K., Henderson, J., Lu, W., & Howard, B. V. (2003). Insulin resistance, the metabolic syndrome, and risk of incident cardiovascular disease in nondiabetic American Indians: the Strong Heart Study. Diabetes care, 26(3), 861-867.

39.   Halberg, N., Henriksen, M., Söderhamn, N., Stallknecht, B., Ploug, T., Schjerling, P., & Dela, F. (2005). Effect of intermittent fasting and refeeding on insulin action in healthy men. Journal of applied physiology, 99(6), 2128-2136.

40.   Safdie, F. M., Dorff, T., Quinn, D., Fontana, L., Wei, M., Lee, C., ... & Longo, V. D. (2009). Fasting and cancer treatment in humans: A case series report. Aging (Albany NY), 1(12), 988.

41.   Di Biase, S., Lee, C., Brandhorst, S., Manes, B., Buono, R., Cheng, C. W., ... & Morgan, T. E. (2016). Fasting-mimicking diet reduces HO-1 to promote T cell-mediated tumor cytotoxicity. Cancer cell, 30(1), 136-146.

42.   Mattson, M. P. (2005). Energy intake, meal frequency, and health: a neurobiological perspective. Annu. Rev. Nutr., 25, 237-260.

43.   Duan, W., Guo, Z., Jiang, H., Ware, M., Li, X. J., & Mattson, M. P. (2003). Dietary restriction normalizes glucose metabolism and BDNF levels, slows disease progression, and increases survival in huntingtin mutant mice. Proceedings of the National Academy of Sciences, 100(5), 2911-2916.

44.   Lee, J., Duan, W., & Mattson, M. P. (2002). Evidence that brain-derived neurotrophic factor is required for basal neurogenesis and mediates, in part, the enhancement of neurogenesis by dietary restriction in the hippocampus of adult

mice. Journal of neurochemistry, 82(6), 1367-1375.

45.   Reusens, B., & Remacle, C. (2001). Intergenerational effect of an adverse intrauterine environment on perturbation of glucose metabolism. Twin Research and Human Genetics, 4(5), 406-411.

46.   Lindsay, R. M. (1994). Neurotrophins and receptors. In Progress in brain research (Vol. 103, pp. 3-14). Elsevier.

47.   Aly, S. M. (2014). Role of intermittent fasting on improving health and reducing diseases. International journal of health sciences, 8(3).

48.   Kacimi, S., Ref'at, A., Fararjeh, M. A., Bustanji, Y. K., Mohammad, M. K., & Salem, M. L. (2012). Intermittent fasting during Ramadan attenuates proinflammatory cytokines and immune cells in healthy subjects. Nutrition research, 32(12), 947-955.

Disclaimer

The information contained in **"Intermittent Fasting – How To Easily Lose Weight, Keep It Off And Improve Your Health,"** and its components, is meant to serve as a comprehensive collection of strategies that the author of this eBook has done research about. Summaries, strategies, tips and tricks are only recommendations by the author, and reading this eBook will not guarantee that one's results will exactly mirror the author's results.

The author of this Ebook has made all reasonable efforts to provide current and accurate information for the readers of this eBook. The author and its associates will not be held liable for any unintentional errors or omissions that may be found.

The material in the Ebook may include information by third parties. Third party materials comprise of opinions expressed by their owners. As such, the author of this eBook does not assume responsibility or liability for any third party material or opinions.

The publication of third party material does not constitute the author's guarantee of any information, products, services, or opinions contained within third party material. Use of third party material does not guarantee that your results will mirror our results. Publication of such third party material is simply a recommendation and expression of the author's own opinion of that material.

Whether because of the progression of the Internet, or the unforeseen changes in company policy and editorial submission guidelines, what is stated as fact at the time of this writing may become outdated or inapplicable later.

www.ingramcontent.com/pod-product-compliance
Lightning Source LLC
LaVergne TN
LVHW020048270625
814836LV00007B/306